1st Edition

Cover Tattoo Cross Art by Renee Mandrake

Infinite Infinites, in Infinite Ways, and at Infinite Levels; Jesus Lead the Way!

A Novella by Shawn Michael Scibelli

Contents

Anything is Possible!

Living life in this 21st century is already full of comforts, luxury goods and services, people willing to help in many ways, easily accessible plentitudes of information, many systems for control (socially, politically, economically, etc.), and establishments of all kinds (some for the better and others for the worse of course). I, however, would very much love to believe that we are all overall tending to still push the envelopes on all fronts of progress towards improving our world and collective existence infinitely more!

Through group thinking, competitive power hierarchies, consciousness, spirit, energy, frequency, vibration, etc. we are all probably connected on at least some levels. So as long as we continue to believe, imagine, and put in the work/effort we can definitely push those envelopes collectively and individually to our desires. This is because ultimately anything is possible despite the way that everything is currently!

There is this particular type of way of existence, however, where things may seem so far out of reach, hopeless, depressing, and boring which seems to befall on those of us who choose to let it or due to a lack of will, imagination, etc. and I feel as well as know that it is such a great and too common of an obstacle that we must learn to adapt to overcome as human-beings if we are to truly take our collective and individual existences to that next level! However, those times when we are "down and out" are not necessarily bad overall either since they can lead to a lot of personal growth and are also just as influential of course in making us who we are today. Even loneliness has potentially tremendous benefits such as creating an opening for "solo levelling" or self-improvement. Many famous/popular, happy, and fulfilled people seek such lonely times out and go as far as to pay to be secluded in a dark, very basic, and secluded living space on some distant nature retreat camp. Furthermore, we all need to know ourselves and stay true to who we are. Each one of us is different of course and will go through our own journeys obviously in order to further discover more about our own potentially infinitely deep souls and consciousnesses. One of the most famous sayings in Ancient times that many may not be aware of is: "Temest nosce", which from Latin translates to "Know thyself". I recall it was on the top entranceway to some Ancient religion's temple, for example, as a main point to be expressed before entry of course. Some people may go through life not understanding the grave importance of this aspect of existence or take poor advice on the lines of faking it until you make it or just be like the others you see whether it be really who they are or some brain washing agenda tracing its routes to a planned psychological operation for social control i.e. T.V. and news potentially with its great power of being able to control the masses opinions and understanding of their current reality in our society. One should understand though that when you're not staying true to yourself a.k.a. being fake, you're hurting yourself in many ways and on many levels. Overall though you are basically becoming a zombie, a welcome mat to someone or something else and almost like basically being nothing at all. For when you are being yourself, it is truly you that is living life and therefore most alive!

Returning to the prior thoughts about that way of existence where one may find themselves feeling hopeless, bored, depressed, etc., I believe that despite how they can lead to many benefits that there is a particular couple of results that I am strongly opposed to. The first is a rhythmic just going through the motions, barely alive spiritually, consciously, and mentally on some levels of being truly awake/aware, as well as without self-empowerment, and without powerful motivation or at least without a positive outlook on the future. It can be very easy at times to fall prey to this rhythmic or repetitive daily existence where you can feel almost more like a robot than human. Beyond that basicness though it goes much deeper to the way that you're consciously experiencing your life. Are you not living in the present moment and just thinking about the same things over and over while not striving for any positive changes or improvement or using your amazingly powerful imagination to attain new levels of spiritual empowerment, new dreams to accomplish, or seriously planning your way to and working towards living your best life? At the very least you should always try and stay in the moment even during bad, dull, or seemingly repetitive experiences. Even the same river that is crossed at the same place is different the next time you cross it, down to a molecular, atomic, and sub-atomic level, etc., and its overall vibe and energy which you changed and/or others as well when you first crossed it and potentially in infinite other ways and at infinite varying levels. Even if certain levels and ways seem unattainable or able to be maxed out, they aren't or at least have the infinite potential to not be if the envelope is pushed in some new or different way or level or if the universe itself changed. Again ultimately anything is possible but yes, of course, the way things are is the way they currently are! Furthermore, to expand on this, this is all to say that while there are maybe only so many things (limited amount), existing in only so many ways (limited amount of ways), and at only so many varying levels that are actually in existence and/or currently possible which all combined makes this/our universe the way that it is overall; ultimately there are infinite possibilities possible (if not currently in this universe until maybe they are, then maybe in another, etc.) which can be further described (from my own perspective of categorizing at least) as infinite infinites (infinite different things/whatever/whoever), existing in possibly infinite different ways, and at possibly infinite different, varying levels. Anything that's imagined including things, ways, levels, or whatever else that's impossible currently can still exist, or come into existence, or be done still when and if the impossible changes to become possible, the impossible is done any way (doing the impossible) because ultimately anything is possible (like for God in the Holy Bible, for example), and/or because it could be possible in a different universe, other place, other time line, or whatever other imaginable varying world/reality. Regardless of all of this though, ultimately the way that our universe is currently is very beautiful and incredibly amazing thanks to God and/or gods/aliens and/or our own collective consciousness (nobody truly knows what consciousness is or where it comes from ultimately despite what they may claim), and/or whatever you believe in as a greater power or powers of consciousness, etc. Furthermore by at least staying in the present moment we can learn from our mistakes much better/easier and focus on letting it sink in in order to motivate you to manifest a better reality and/or change whatever it is or way that caused you to have a bad experience in your life and to prevent and understand it better of course.

Just as we can all rise and improve, however, we can also always fall and get worse so it is up to you and the people close to you to keep up the positive momentum or spirit. This brings me to the second result which I'm concerned with and that is fear itself. Most people are pretty aware of course of its great sway and effects on their reality. It can be so damaging to let fear control you or society in general as it often can become so unhinged leading to a potential downward spiral of madness chasing off an over-hyped agitation/concern.

A lot of times throughout my life and especially recently I've found meditation to be the best medicine for remedying this in general; as one can really hone in on and think super clearly about their thoughts uninterrupted and with greater focus compared to being distracted or multitasking such as when driving your vehicle at the same time. I also strongly believe that people should also focus more on caring about their own life, actions, thoughts, and even vibe that's projected outward on others and the world. For all we know, reincarnation is real and everything from your current existence will carry over and affect any future existences in this realm and/or others i.e. the spiritual world (this I do believe). At the very least, it may be of great benefit in many ways to adopt such beliefs as people would probably care more about everything especially with the understanding of one of the greatest truths of all that ultimately anything is possible so you can most definitely achieve your greatest dreams somehow, someway in this life or the next! Now for those of us who choose to follow Jesus Christ as the Son of God and have read the *Holy Bible* (I read the King James version) we can recall His words in saying that anything is possible with God! This was in a conversation He had with a rich man wondering about his prospects for getting into Heaven and Jesus' response was that it would be like trying to fit a camel through a pinhole which is normally impossible of course but with God, He said, anything is possible (*Holy Bible*, 2016)!

Rising

I remember a time in my life which was years ago just before I had felt compelled to read a book called *Thirsty for God: A Brief History of Christian Spirituality*, by Bradley P. Holt, and then the *Holy Bible* itself shortly thereafter. It was a lonelier, depressing time but still there was plenty of hope and light. I didn't have many friends; I was new to the real world, post-college life yet I still had a couple of really great ones which is probably true for many others especially in this day and age. This was also all I probably really needed anyway looking back now. Anyway, I recall a time when a friend and I had partied the prior night, drinking and smoking some cannabis. I felt sober the next day but I also felt really happy overall and content with the present moment in that I believed that thanks to God somehow everything would work out in the end for the best. Beyond that though, I somehow convinced myself to let go of all fears, anxieties, etc. in order to just experience the present moment, to live and breathe freely, staying completely true to myself. I remember driving with the windows down, feeling the air surround, reflect off of, and pass through my fingers as I stuck my hand out. I was also looking but not simply just looking. I was really taking in experiences, appreciating, and remembering all the buildings, people, scenery, etc. as I passed by. It was all so much more magical, powerful, and exciting to experience life this way (like stopping to smell the roses as it's said often or feeling the rain on your skin). Moreso I felt like I was experiencing the presence of God in the sense that I was actively seeking him out to say the least w/ strong belief and I came up with a seemingly perfect way of thinking about this new found way of experiencing reality. I would think to myself: breathe, meditate, and remember the way. Breathing deeply and especially consciously with great focus, I found, brought me into a better state of mind overall and with a better capacity to then focus on living in the present in order to accomplish the other two ideas of meditating and thinking about/remembering that new found way of living and experiencing my own existence in this amazingly cool world we live in. Even if you're not currently in a good place physically, spiritually, mentally, etc., you can still stay positive and always have hope for a better future in understanding and believing the truth that ultimately anything is possible so things can and will get better! I will return to these newly found ideas that I discovered but I feel that I must first fully explain not only the importance of this truth but the realization and break down of the understanding of what is an essential truth to me and how it's existence can be witnessed and proven.

It all starts with how this all started, for all of us of course. There are so many so called experts (paid shills pushing an agenda or serious intellectuals critically thinking) or actual scientists doing experiments and discovering truths about our reality through the actual scientific proven method of hypothesizing, experimenting, forming a theory, and testing it by comparing results with a control, etc. Of the main stream theories, however, there is the one known as The Big Bang Theory which has significantly grown in popularity over the years and is widely accepted. Though it may or may not be true; no one can say for sure of course right now based on the available facts, evidence, etc. However it all actually did start though for our particular universe, one truth seems to be self-evident: it's all things, consciousness, spirit, etc. that are in existence instead of or coming out of nothing. It is a very magical and truly amazing concept to grasp that that is the case. Whether everything and everyone came magically out of nothingness or has just simply always been (without the idea/concept of time which some say doesn't actually exist in our universe anyway) instead of there being nothing, both are equally possible and both must be true at the same time since you could always have a something that has always been in existence out of nothingness that could have the quality or ability to be able to bring something, anything into existence or the opposite where a something that came to be out of nothingness creates something that can change everything including itself of course so that it has always been (rewriting and/or deleting the past entirely). Perhaps the greatest realization of all of this though is that any of these things that are existing in existence and came to be instead of and/or out of nothing could have been anything else that you can imagine and even that which you cannot yet (imagination is the truer sign of intelligence compared to knowledge and there are infinite levels of intelligence possible). This becomes true and self-evident beginning with when we examine the very definition of there being nothing or absolute nothingness which is of course there being no thing or anyone at all including a universe or thing with a trait or physical laws that govern it.

Without any laws or physics or anything at all to govern what is or will be; there cannot be determination as to what will be or has been unless it was brought forth, either intentionally or not, from something or someone else existing instead of or out of nothing. Furthermore, no rules inside absolute nothingness means if something came to be or will become something or someone out of it; then it could very well have been or will be anything at all. In other words and to expand upon that further: there are no rules inside nothing where anything magically can come to be and thereby no law(s) or restriction(s) or anything else to forcibly determine what that something will be and there are infinite possibilities as to what can be imagined to be and therefore potentially exist (a something, someone, anything at all). Also, even though there are the laws of conservation of mass and energy whereby it's stated that no mass or energy can be created or destroyed; that is just the way it is currently in our universe and thankfully so. However, other universes within our multiverse or in a different one potentially infinitely beyond and completely separated from our own may have different laws whereby matter could be created and/or destroyed since there are no rules or laws inside absolute nothingness whereby anything could have come to be someway or another including different universes with different physics, laws, etc. Think about how truly awe-inspiring, incredible, and powerful all of this is to realize. We should all be infinitely more grateful and appreciative of our own existence! You may not have existed and there are those who do not you could say from a possibility perspective; so praise God that you do!

Also, even if everything exists instead of and not out of nothing, it still holds true that where there's no rules, laws of nature, physics, etc. there are infinite possibilities as to what can be out there already instead of nothing including that something or someone that can create anything it imagines (for whatever reasons) out of nothing. Or even just due to there being different rules, physics, laws of nature, or whatever governing force in a different universe or even multiverse full of entirely different universes; there could be anything and everything else imaginable somewhere out there. Furthermore, maybe there are different multiverses and/or universes or whatever else that's completely separated from ours due to it existing in an entirely different realm, spatial place, dimension, or just broken off completely from ours and separated with a layer of space of nothingness in between so that it's entirely undetectable and doesn't interact or affect ours at all. Or maybe there could just be the inability for the two worlds to collide and/or interact due to a lack of relationship in the sense that they're so incompatible and uniquely different for whatever other reason that they could occupy the same space and overlap but not affect each other at all yet still with the possibility of them changing in order to interact always there potentially as well. Two different worlds colliding is a scary thought but it could also introduce great positive changes as well potentially. Nonetheless God can do anything so I believe we shouldn't have fear on these or any such matters ultimately.

Breathe, Meditate, Remember the Way!

ow finally returning back to those two newly found ideas of meditating and remembering/following the way, I believe that meditating is an especially powerful tool that I discovered and only really started using within the past few years. The meditation I am referring to (because there are so many different styles, techniques, etc.) is basically and put as simply as I would like to describe it: doing your very best to stop thinking about everything and only letting those fleeting, present moment thoughts that have to do only with what is actually happening now in front of you to occur and staying in the present moment with all of your conscious being, taking everything (the good and the bad) in but focusing more on the good of course while reminding yourself every once in awhile of all the amazing opportunities possible (anything) and the magical truth of being someone alive now (how strange it is to be anything at all). Also the key to a successful meditation in this way is to actually remember and follow that way that is all about being fearlessly in the moment and trusting in God as your savior who will be there for you against all odds and evils. The fear must be overcome and driven out as it will take you over, causing your spirit to freeze up and lead you down a dark spiral where it can be so easy to stop being yourself, living freely and consciously true to yourself. Also of course because your goal really ultimately should be to bring about self love, happiness, improvement in all ways, and becoming more alive and closer to God with a greater appreciation and thrill of living life to the fullest!

Another technique of meditation, which I invented on my own, comes from the idea that we as humans do not think nor do we have the ability to be able to think truly randomly because it is not good for survival with the way that our world has been overall throughout our evolution. Furthermore, our thoughts are only somewhat random, influenced by the current state of our brain, mood, environment, fatigue, our prior experiences, etc. So while sometimes our thoughts may seem random at times, they're not truly random as our brain operates as a causal system whereby which every thought comes from prior brain activity which was formed by biology, emotion, perception, and memory. This is why even seemingly random thoughts are actually in fact unpredictable but not truly random because they have a chain of causes. It is because of all of this that our brains generate outputs from internal processing (a recalled memory or something that was observed in your environment visually, etc.) as opposed to a source of true randomness such as a truly random number generator using random electronic noise or radioactive decay. We operate our brains from this causal system which is based upon our past experiences and our sometimes own self-formed patterns of thought which leads to us having our biased, unpredictable thinking. As an example, even if you attempted to think up some totally random word, you would instead make up words from partial themes, meanings, of your own language, etc. but nothing truly random and without pattern or influence from recent thoughts, words you already know, subconscious association, etc. To entertain a fun thought experiment since anything is possible, a human could achieve the ability of being able to think truly randomly naturally if they were able to remove or override internal cognitive bias and replace it with the utilization of a source capable of generating physical randomness which has a mapping system that then avoids human choice during selection and finally is read without filtering. Thus all in all, ultimately this way and technique of meditating that I'm about to describe in detail is basically a thought experiment in and of itself which may or may not actually work but nonetheless might be interesting to study the short and long term effects of which also may or may not be useful and positively productive. So then this is one work around which I thought of for people who would like to try meditating in randomness as a potentially and hypothetically (admittedly, I've no idea and haven't studied this much at all) useful way of achieving a breakthrough break away from their normal, habitual cycles and state of mind, seemingly or potentially even somewhat maybe (maybe not) fated bad reality, thinking loops of repeated dwelling or thinking about the same things or in the same way constantly, just out of curiosity or interest in a uniquely new method, and/or boredom of other meditations. With an AI tool such as ChatGPT and a truly random number generator such as the website: "random.org", you can generate random numbers and then have ChatGPT quickly and easily translate that random small batch of numbers into words or at least nonsensical attempts for words (aka random letters grouped together). One technique is generating numbers 1-26 for the amount of letters in the alphabet and then teaching the AI to subsequently recognize the code (for example, a=1, b=2, c=3, d=4, etc.) to decode after relaying the combo of numbers through the AI. Next you can then repeat the random combo of letters/word, formed by the AI, in your head and think about it briefly in silent meditation in terms of things such as what that word may mean to you or make you think of or just think on it exactly for whatever that "word" might be even if it it's not a real word: for example "ctsrkwl" might make you think cats are cool which is of course a random thought you may not have thought without utilizing these tools. You can also go without ChatGPT and just figure out what the words are based on whatever code you formulate in your mind (depends on how you want to meditate i.e. with more or less thinking) or even just the numbers themselves so as to not assign any bias at all to whatever those randomly generated numerical outputs happened to be which were obtained perhaps potentially much easier than other natural forms of randomness which maybe can be obtained in nature itself on our planet or through our daily lives, etc (OpenAI, 2026).

The next topic I wanted to bring attention to is how we'll all face great adversity, basically always in our own personal pursuits of happiness of course where there is competition (competition can of course be very good and healthy too) everywhere attempting to do the same living under seemingly finite resources. This sparks a lot of fear, anger, and resentment towards each other and the truth is that that's okay too since there is such thing as good, healthy fear that does make the world a better place when we are all more fearful and as a result more careful about certain things such as artificial intelligence technology growing at such increasingly rapid rates in its improvement.

Anger too can help spark a lot of personal growth, introspection, and be an overall great source of motivation at times. However, some say that infinite free energy has already been discovered (Nikola Tesla rumors for example) but true or not there always could be more of anything out there in the infinite great beyond (even beyond our own universe, in different universes, multiverses, etc.) Now on the flip side of course, thinking about things from perhaps a more realistic viewpoint, if we are not able to somehow figure out how to obtain what we need close by (our planet, solar system, galaxy, universe, etc.) or at least enough of it then yes, indeed we could very well find it beyond our current place but traveling great distances may require great amounts of energy or work or if none of those then at least great risk as one ventures out deeper and deeper into the infinite unknown.

The concept of friendly competition, in my opinion, is the ideal and most suitable for us to all live in harmony and with greater and greater happiness as we all grow and collectively improve our own lives, each others' lives, and the world at large. Indeed of course striving to be better in whatever way and attaining whatever level pushes us to go beyond our previous limits and attain new ones as we make and keep to our goals or feel a sense of motivation. On that note though, I have personally found that staying disciplined has been able to keep me most on track for my own goals as I haven't always felt motivated on long term goals especially but discipline ensures the necessary consistency which is so key to success in goals such as training to run your first marathon or losing weight. Still, inspiring motivation in myself for whatever cause or goal has been extremely beneficial too and everyone is different in terms of what keeps them going and from where they draw their own inspiration or source of energy to do that.

For some it might help to just start with smaller goals and focus on these or on enjoying the journey itself in whatever ways you can creatively come up with such as listening to music or a podcast or multitasking with anything else you might be able to really enjoy like playing video games on a treadmill. Although I personally hate treadmills and would always much rather run outside enjoying the beautiful scenes, weather, fresh air, feeling the more real experience of it all and listening to music which helps inspire me tremendously and makes so many mundane or other tasks much more doable and enjoyable even. I'm actually honestly listening to music as I write this!

Competition under the right conditions itself can be very enjoyable for probably most of us and especially those of us with a competitor spirit (definitely me). Those unfavorable conditions though when things get so out of whack in terms of fairness or gross injustice such as enslavement of a conquered people with horrendous conditions can create such a terrible existence for many that it may even get close to a point of being almost like a form of hell on earth. Enslavement that is hidden and tremendous gaps between the wealthy have and have nots even goes on today and while it is great to reap your own rewards for what you do; there are many that may simply inherit great wealth and power of course which they may sometimes not actually possibly and seemingly deserve. Some could maybe just be members of what some call the lucky sperm club. However, who actually knows how much of it is just luck or actual deserving fate, placement by God, or a higher power, etc.? It's all possible but ultimately we should all strive to make the world better or at least leave it a little bit better from when you came into it in whatever ways you can.

There is absolutely great power, wealth, enjoyment, fun, etc. to be experienced and received as well, however, when rising together as a group of consciousnesses/people as opposed to just being out for your own personal gain always. Sometimes a group of people may create a hellish existence for many to experience on earth or things may seem to devolve into chaos or go backwards in many ways on great progress we made as a whole society which of course is terribly unfortunate. While I would like to remain positive about all of that and hope that most people would not want to live in a form of hell on earth, there is a lot of evil present in our world obviously with many evil, cold, and cruel people only out to please themselves (sociopaths, psychopaths, etc.). Instead of the opposite it would be great if we all aimed to collectively improve our world. Many may fear change, however of course or may just not care as long as only their own ambitions are fulfilled or may just not believe and understand that ultimately anything is possible and there are no limits to how much better things could be and the progress we could all make rising together!

Now let's think about the way that some things are in reality right now that maybe have a lot of great benefits to them but I personally believe we ought to be at least more aware of and responsible with especially as they progress to a higher level in some ways. I'll start with a scenario of a typical American's life and break down the aspects of what I'm thinking of in relation to the above notion. So this guy named Bill is a regular guy who works at an investment firm for his regular 9-5, 5 days a week job. Do you know what Bill does at work? He stares at a screen inside his cubicle like the main character, Neo, in *The Matrix* movie (The Wachowskis, 1999).

His whole day begins with him waking up inside his house which actually isn't really his, it's someone else's who he rents a small tight studio room from. It's basically just a box big enough for his bed, a dresser, night stand, and his beloved 52 inch 3D TV. After he wakes he's practically right off to work in his speedy little green, ugly, box-like smart car that hopefully will make a significant enough of a difference to save the planet through a reduced carbon footprint (without better future carbon removal and sequestration technologies, for example, etc.).

The ugly green box on wheels does the job very efficiently though getting him to his other box that is his cubicle at work which he might as well be chained to for all the time he slaves away for basically just enough scraps of wealth to feed himself, his box master (I mean landlord), that actually mostly coal powered box on wheels (currently the origin of the vast majority of the electricity generated) which actually these days of his life in year 2105 costs quite a decent chunk of his paycheck to pay off the sizeable loan which was taken out for it, and stay relevant with the newest hand-held pocket screen and the next better screen T.V. for home. He dreams that maybe he'll save up enough for a bigger or better located box (I mean house) of his own someday with a front or backyard which is currently well beyond his pay grade in the big city where he works. So let's break down Bill's life into the recognizably perhaps pathetic in some people's opinions (my own opinion included) borderline enslaving pattern that it is: he works at that cubicle box where he stares at a screen all day in order to maybe someday afford a cooler box on wheels to take him back to his self-owned home box all the while he's glaring down at his pocket sized screen for just a gasp of some sort of quick fix of dopamine from someone impressing him with their fantastical existence that he can only dream of attaining (and maybe it is something he could actually very easily obtain like a trip to a tropical beach that shouldn't actually be such a restricted and extremely expensive experience if it weren't for the distance, threat of danger vs safe tourist only vacation hotspot hotel and resort area, and highly overpriced food and amenities forced on the non-locals). This matrix of boxes and screens that increasingly seems to takeover people's lives in our modern existence, especially in the big city, is not always a bad thing as there are many benefits such as ease of entertainment, safety, reliable commuting, easygoing lifestyles, etc. but overall I think it is important to recognize real experiences from fake or metaverse ones, existing vs living life to the fullest, true progress vs progress in a metaverse or artificially created worlds, and the values learned from dystopian extremes on these concepts as seen in *The Matrix* and the other films of that trilogy for example (The Wachowskis, 1999).

The Real World

Yes, our real world can seem difficult, more dangerous than playing that addictive MMORPG game which doesn't have real consequences, and very unfair at times especially when all the wealth and power is concentrated into the hands of a select few coined the "1%'ers," etc. but we must all remember that ultimately anything is possible and we all truly can achieve our dreams one way or another, this life or the next, somewhere, somehow, and through infinity and beyond (hopefully not to sound too corny like a Buzz Lightyear from *Toy Story*)(Lasseter, 1995)! Also, technically on the flip side of things it is interesting to think about the metaverse, the idea of a matrix or simulated reality from the perspective of all things being connected. Going back to there being positives to take away from all of these ideas, concepts, and thinking about reality vs artificially created realities; even the most seemingly fake realities such as what you dream at night are in some way and at some level connected to this real world experience that we live and breathe in each day. Literally and figuratively the dreams affect your real world in the sense that even your thoughts matter and everything else (not just physical actual matter in the literal sense of the word and definition) matters too! Supposedly as some say and believe, everything in this Universe that we call home (the way it is in reality of course) can be classified as sourcing from energy and/or electromagnetic radiation (the physical), spirit, consciousness, and other whatever that we do not understand such as dark matter and dark energy (which apparently isn't actually energy according to some astrophysical theorists).

Now the ways in which all of this stuff and we consciousnesses existing in human or other alien forms (I'm sure there are other intelligent or not beings and forms of life existing in all sorts of strange ways to us, i.e. plants, and other unknown life forms) are probably connected; could be on some level so as to bring about real change, cause and effect, etc. from perhaps any interactions even if only on a microscopic, atomic, subatomic, metaphysical, or even in spiritual ways which we cannot understand. In terms of the realistic impact however, it could be so very, very tiny of course as to be considered basically negligible but it is still something which ultimately means it matters. Furthermore, even in what is my opinion of a maybe bad or good type of unknown simulation or dystopian perspectives of such i.e. *The Matrix* film; there could always be an undertone, connection of a sort, and/or valuable relationship which is possible in terms of such a world or existence's relation to a "realer" or mega (above the meta level for example or a higher level or layer) world above it. (The Wachowskis, 1999). I think it's also fascinating to think about and imagine computer systems that run on entirely different number systems outside of the commonly used, standard system of 0's and 1's such as ternary which has 0's, 1's, and 2's or one that is mapped as having 0's, 1's, 2's, 3's, 4's, and 5's (could potentially, possibly have infinitely more as well or use letters or symbols like hieroglyphics to represent some other utilizations of a different kind of energy) whereby which: 0 = off, 1 = very, very low voltage, 2 = very low voltage, 3 = low voltage, 4 = medium voltage, and 5 = high voltage.

All the so called fake worlds of course such as a kid's video game still exist in our literal real world in some way and at some level even if it's seen from the simple perspective of just being a show of lights. That is not to say that a video game is real obviously but simply the obvious truth that it does have real impacts and actually if what some believe to be true, that our world's physical nature is actually light energy more than anything at the actual source level of electromagnetic radiation, then maybe even more real than some realize. Though those lights dancing on the usual T.V. screen are 2-D as they appear and are of course; it is interesting to think about and realize how despite an alive being only seeing essentially the tally mark for the number one if they were to experience life in a 2-D world, even the smallest line if zoomed in close enough onto can appear as a big rectangle. This means that since technically something can be zoomed in on an infinite amount of times and levels down past its microscopic makeup, atomically, and beyond until the limits of this particular universe (entropy) if there are any, are reached, even light particles for example displaying in a 2D world can possibly evolve into 3D essentially through such an increased magnification as seen from within that 2D perspective. I think it's amazing and cool to become aware of that possibility and connection between the 2D and 3D worlds.

Shining another light and actually a positive vision on that day to day repetitive "rat race", corporate American complex, feeling sometimes like you're trapped where you are maybe type of an existence or just another number/cog in a machine and that overall subsequential struggle of our 21st century lifestyles that some of us may very unfortunately and seemingly more easily fall victim to (especially during and as a result of the horrific lockdowns of the world basically from 2020-2021); we can all do so much to change things both individually and collectively. Individually, I'm talking about doing things such as getting outside like you took a lesson from Henry David Thoreau; going for a hike and/or camping trip for example and enjoying every bit of that natural scenery, vibing along your path with every step upon the rocks, pebbles, and through the streams of Mother Earth and nature as you progress forwards along your physical, spiritual, and energetic changing, building, and influencing journey of living life.

Also, if you find (and you probably will) that many people nowadays around you and your community at large are more socially shy, awkward, isolationist, and reclusive to their homes of comfort, you can still get out as much as you can, summoning every bit of confidence and energy to make that change of bringing about a more social and interactive face to face existence. For every downfall that this new technology has created with so much addiction to screen time, we have at least enabled a very easy way to reach out to others so instantly and with that many cyber realms also for communicating with, planning, and initiating meet ups for in "real life" for those like-minded souls out there who would like to collectively make a difference. We all really (as corny as it sounds) need to start being the positive change in the world that we want to see instead of waiting for things to change around us.

Things could get infinitely better for all of us and I mean that literally in the sense that there really are no limits to improving, being happier, loving more and more deeply, and enjoying life infinitely more through whatever is fun, a great experience, etc. for you. The truth is that none of us truly knows how deep our world goes inwards and of course outward. There is the defined scientifically measurable entropy or physical extents of which any object has in terms of its levels/layers of quantifiable characteristics observably impacting the physical world and providing data for us to collect and measure numerically and mathematically, however, of course. Though this doesn't necessarily cover everything especially if as some have hypothesized that everything in our world may actually be pure consciousness which just as a soul can be infinitely deep, consciousness can be too!

The Supernatural

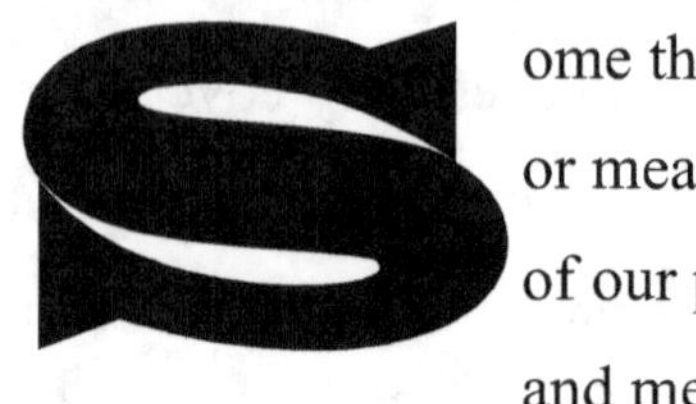ome things just aren't visible or measurable for us with all of our physical technologies and measuring objects at our disposal. I do believe that the "spirit world" is very real as do many others and there is a lot of proof of its existence actually despite all of the difficulty in physically and scientifically observing it. For example, there are many who have experienced super-natural occurrences like a near death experience coupled with an out of body experience where they very seemingly observe a fragment of the after-life such as seeing their own body or a spiritual world.

I myself have experienced what I at least believed to be something from beyond the known physical realm in the sense that it may have been more spiritual, religious (being from God), and miraculous or supernatural. That was the very memorable dream I had one night which felt very realistic and powerful to me. I was inside a church floating above and moving around to different perspectives as I observed Jesus Christ sitting on the floor, holding hands with the children around him, forming a cross together as they all sat in rows of two with Jesus on the right side, at the end, holding hands with the child next to him as Satan was trying desperately to no avail to come through the floor below to reach them. This dream of Jesus was one of maybe three I recall in my life with the other two very vaguely remembered at all making it that much more memorable, meaningful, and powerful to me as mentioned before.

This dream also seemed to be at least markedly somewhat coincidental to me as I recall all of the child abuse that had been all over the news and discussed often as having occurred so terribly and rampantly throughout the Christian churches world-wide and was really being uncovered for many through many mainstream reporting outlets with a lot of direct evidence and witnesses first-hand and what not coming forward. I chose to believe that if God was possibly communicating to me through this dream then He was telling me that He was with the children and was protecting them from the satanic pedophiles of the world. Furthermore, just as Jesus had said that it would be better that a millstone should hang from the necks of those who abuse children; I believe that at the very least these evil abusers will be punished in

Hell. Then later the following day the Notre Dame spire went up in flames which made me wonder if that correlated at all to the dream and beliefs I had about it. Was God punishing "the church" for all of the abuse it had willfully ignored for so long and even contributed to?

There was a lot of abuse reported in the Christian churches in France and around the world sadly. What if this was God's way of getting our attention to what was going on in His churches and wanted us to cleanse and rebuild like the Flood had done before. God had said that He wouldn't flood the world again but that the next time it would be by fire and then a new Earth would be created for the righteous, good souls, and believers to start anew and live better. After the dream that I had, I experienced an interesting, surprising, and quite strange phenomena of my smoke detector going off repeatedly for a couple years now, randomly (except for it happening again a few days after writing about this) and at all three of the residences that I lived at and moved to despite the batteries being changed and detectors being replaced (it just kept happening). These experiences made me think that maybe God was trying to message me about the dream, wanting to remind me about it, and spread the word about it but of course I have no idea still for sure what it was all about. I'm honestly of course just making assumptions about what I'd like to believe.

When I was in fifth grade I remember feeling very sick with belly aches for awhile until I eventually was diagnosed (and very possibly inaccurately) with Crohn's disease. Maybe it could be true as some in more recent times have wondered and suggested that Crohn's, Celiac's, and the increasingly more common allergies, autoimmune, and chronic illnesses are actually caused by vaccines and other man-made pollutants throughout our current modern environment. Despite all of this I managed to heal so very seemingly completely, starting from a few years ago when the whole pandemic lockdown occurred preventing many from seeing Dr.'s in person unless for emergencies for a short time which was when I actually decided to try and take a more natural route to my health and eventually came off all of my prescription drugs.

I started focusing on my mental, spiritual, physical health, etc. doing things such as meditating more, eating way healthier (all organic, non-GMO, etc.) praying more to God, reading the *Holy Bible*, running, lifting, swimming, using the sauna to clear my body of toxins along with lemons in my drinking water, making healthy plant smoothies, and more. I even hiked up Mt. Washington in the winter which wasn't even really hiking at some points where already steep cliffs were packed and filled in with a lot of snow and ice which made them even steeper of course and almost vertically straight up walls which required climbing with my ice axe. All in all the hike out and back is a challenging 8 miles and felt almost as challenging as running my first marathon on a flat, paved road, and on a sunny, warm day. I also accomplished that massive running goal after going fully clean and taking my health and overall care of my body, mind, etc. more seriously.

Furthermore, I was able to accomplish two other major athletic, physical goals of mine: run a sub-six minute mile and bench press 225 lbs. (while only weighing 135 lbs. at the time which is considered beyond advanced and around the elite level according to some sources I remember seeing online). To put this all into perspective, Crohn's can be a deadly disease which can cause you to not be able to absorb nutrients so easily and have chronic inflammation, which in turn causes a lot of difficult to manage symptoms such as feeling very tired/weak and stomach cramps/pain among others. Not trying to brag too much here but these were all such massive accomplishments made after going all natural/organic with my healing journey that I never would have dreamed of doing someday back before all of this when I struggled so much with just a simple 5km run and had those symptoms which praise the Lord I don't have currently and haven't for about 4 years now. I never took any of this for granted though and will be the first to admit that things could change in an instant and just as I rose up so to speak, I know I could fall. I'm only human but I will always do my best to at least keep being an inspiration to others out there that may be going through a similar battle and maybe could appreciate that reminder that they too can do it.

Another supernatural occurrence which humanity can actually witness directly in terms of its clear, vastly out of the ordinary, super awe-inspiring appearance in our physical, worldly realm is the Great Pyramid of Giza and really a lot of other pyramids such as the other two under Orion's belt. It is believed that these three though were once colored with the Great Pyramid of Giza being white with a golden top, one red, and the other black. Just by looking at these in person on the outside it is apparently (I've never been) very amazing to imagine the incredible prowess, skills, and power that was used to build them. However, if you step inside then it is even further amazing when one takes into account some of the much bigger blocks which were somehow lifted into positions higher up on top of other gigantic blocks of limestone. Humanity today apparently is barely able to reconstruct even smaller portions of this and some say our best engineers and cranes wouldn't be able to lift some of the bigger blocks to where they are. So how were these pyramids built is the question to ponder especially when considering that just one stone out of the more than 2 million that were supposedly cut, dragged, and lifted to build the Great Pyramid thousands of years ago is absolutely massive and extremely heavy! There are a bunch of hypotheses that attempt to answer this such as a water hydraulics "volcano-like" system and millions of slaves rolling them over logs. I so far haven't believed any of them personally except for one which is that the blocks were levitated by either super intelligent, powerful, much healthier, and more spiritually connected humans with the assistance of aliens or mostly by aliens. I think that the nearby evidence of quartz crystal structures and mines as well as the ancient, super spiritual sound-healing rooms point towards the possibility that maybe the blocks were able to be levitated by beings that were much more connected to the Earth spiritually, more powerful energetically, at a higher level consciously, etc. or something to the point where perhaps maybe they were able to "magically" lift them with their own conscious energy similar to how "the Force" is used in *Star Wars* (Lucas, 1977). This is just a guess but maybe the quartz and perhaps other crystals were used as a way to amplify their energy so that it could be put to a task such as this which might've been to build an interdimensional portal or pyramid structure which amplifies and/or helps to reawaken a whole big community's individual, personally unique abilities from "raising the collective vibe" so to speak, somehow?

Infinite Infinites, Ways, and Levels

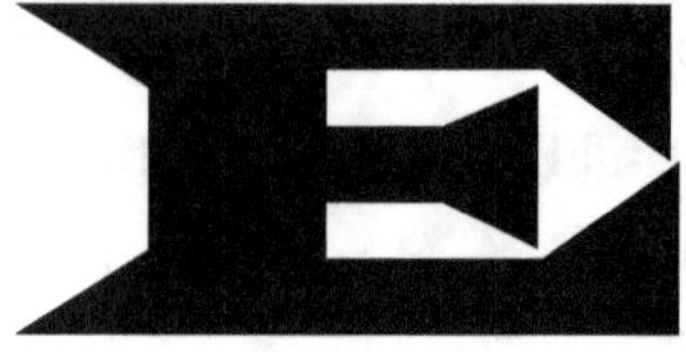xpanding even more and also unpacking this great belief and seemingly probable truth that ultimately anything is possible; we should start with going over and thinking much more deeply about what already is in existence and how it may have come to be. To do that, I've come up with a categorical breakdown which I've placed all things that are of course in existence already. Since technically the unknown and even known things could go on forever in terms of quantity such as existing in what is infinitely beyond the exterior of our very universe and multiverse, I think it makes sense to me to call it all: infinite infinites, existing in infinite ways, and at infinite varying levels. The first of these three descriptive classifications puts literally everything into the category of being a something in existence instead of or out of nothing with the endless possibility of it existing in infinite quantities throughout the infinite known and unknown worlds, universes, multiverses, dimensions, timelines, etc. Furthermore, that is to say that any person,

place, or thing always has the infinite potential to be in existence in infinite quantities elsewhere throughout the infinite beyond. For example, we've all heard of how there could be another person even such as yourself existing in a parallel universe or branched timeline off of our singular universe and these other versions of yourself could be vastly similar or different, etc. and there could be infinite amounts of them. However, I believe we can rest assured in the knowing that they still aren't yourself in the sense of your singular consciousness being that of who you actually are right now because that's the way that consciousness works from at least what I believe and understand to be true which is that of course you are consciously experiencing life as only just yourself here and now in this particular universe as you are. You are obviously also therefore not responsible for the conscious free-will derived decisions of others ultimately including those other consciousnesses living in similar bodies and lives as a version of yourself in other parallel worlds. Furthermore, I believe that even if what some have said is true that we are all one consciousness; we are all separate entities still or parts of that wholly combined one consciousness which can separate while still remaining linked and come back together which is maybe what happens when we pass into the after life (though of course as I also mentioned much earlier: nobody truly knows what consciousness is or where it comes from).

Also, as an example, there could be infinite gold ore in terms of its existing quantities dispersed throughout our universe, multiverse, and even other multiverses infinitely beyond our multiverse of universes. Gold as a form of physical matter also has the potential to come into existence into ours infinitely through infinite ways and at infinite varying levels; especially if just one of many example hypotheses which may be true (but may not be also since nobody knows for sure) that everything is pure consciousness and that consciousness is infinite already in terms of quantity potential and actuality. Regardless, these infinite quantities of infinite different things, each being separated from each other by some distinctive way and at some level such as a single atom of iron as opposed to a single atom of Einsteinium; exist and/or have the potential to exist in our world and/or in other universes, etc. in infinite ways as well. These infinite possible ways (if not in this universe then perhaps in another), to name a few examples, include: the infinite different shapes, infinite different colors, infinite different textures, infinite states of matter (frozen, gas, etc.), etc.

My rule of thumb in regards to this classification is that if it is still considered to be whatever it is, regardless of the differences that make it up or him/her, etc. then it is the same of course at least for classification purposes such as obviously every unique individual (despite race or anything else) still being considered a human-being despite our potentially infinite differences. It never ceases to amaze me; all of the different qualities found naturally amongst similar things that are basically the same as aforementioned in terms of classification such as flowers existing in their infinitely unique ways down to distinct petal shape, size, and color. If we think about that varying way for something to exist such as in different colors, we can imagine the infinitely, continuously varying wavelengths, wave heights, and energies such as light as we know it that would create and allow for the infinite possibilities for infinite other colors to exist that we cannot see currently with the way we human beings are and our current universe is.

However, take for example the hummingbird which has an extra cone for seeing further along that infinite line (going both directions infinitely of course in terms of ultimate potential) of electromagnetic radiation (light) and you have a form of life here on earth that literally does see more colors than we can and actually turtles can too. I think it's really infinitely cool to imagine that there are infinite possible colors and shapes, etc. Actually, believe it or not, I personally know someone who claims to have imagined a color she had not seen before whilst "tripping on a particular someone in the sky with diamonds". Furthermore, like sort of how Albert Einstein talked about relativity with the classically popular example of time moving much more slowly to you when you are sitting on burning hot coals as opposed to having fun partying where time would move much faster, we can also imagine how potentially in other universes, worlds, or existences or forms of life; those much bigger or tinier electromagnetic radiation waves of light, that we either see or cannot yet see as visibly different colors of light, could be relatively more regular, easier, or normal sized to whatever could/would produce them like a star and whoever/whatever else would then process and see them.

Alternatively, there could very possibly be other worlds or universes or multiverses, etc. that either have different colors and properties for where the visible light waves would be for humans in terms of an energy wave's length, height, etc., and position on that numerical line chart of electromagnetic radiation (which since numbers can go on infinitely that line can too of course) or have more commonly occurring different waves or a greater variety of them existing naturally or for them to be much more possible to be in existence. The possibilities really are endless; other universes could have different forms of electromagnetic radiation or something even completely different: a whole different type of energy or something similar but different from energy itself that doesn't exist here in our universe.

These infinite infinites existing in infinite ways as aforementioned also exist at infinite varying levels. We've all probably heard that popular saying: "I'm gonna take things to a whole 'notha level," or something similar which expresses exactly what I'm herein referring to of course. That is to say that just as something such as H2O can exist in a different way here in our universe such as a crystal clear block of ice (let's say 3x3ft for all intensive purposes) it can also have infinite potential levels to it in terms of it's size let's say for a very simplistic, obvious example (infinitely bigger or infinitely smaller potentially maybe in our universe or others of course). A cooler example, pun intended, in my opinion though would be that of a mixed martial arts fighter where you can imagine how there are all different levels of actual proven performance based on varying levels of skills, knowledge in the sport, etc. You can have infinitely higher levels of physical fighting competitive prowess where all fighters are rated numerically by their level of overall potential fighting capabilities or just simply by ranking on a world-wide leaderboard.

This idea of infinite potential levels also can be rather simply exemplified by the physically larger and smaller units of anything. That is to say that just as one could observe the existence of an ultra massive diamond which technically could always be even infinitely bigger still; that diamond has a structure which makes it up to be what it is and that can be traced inward through levels of actual matter. These levels of matter are the potentially infinitely separable and identifiable layers, pieces, and units. For example, we all know how that carbon structure of a diamond can be traced inward to single atoms of carbon but if you go deeper there's the protons, electrons, neutrons; even deeper there's the sub-atomic particles, and even deeper than that nobody knows as far as I'm aware but there's always potential for infinitely smaller particles and (in this universe or another, etc.) layers and thereby levels.

During the Coronavirus pandemic, I had a lot of free time on my hands with basically everything shut down and actually for some time even quite literally everything was closed and we were all locked down inside our homes. With the government enforced shutdown all of us except for essential workers and those who could work from home of course were living this way of having plenty of time to themselves and their loved ones or friends especially with the highly popular and easy ways to connect virtually these days such as Discord chat rooms. I and many others turned to video games for the freedom and entertainment values which were so desired at that time. They're also very fun of course as competitive as they can be as well as at times, especially when played together with friends or new acquaintances you may meet when playing them online together with people from literally all over the world.

I had so much time to just think, play video games, train for running my first marathon, and I was also able to even finish reading the *Holy Bible*. I was playing a number of different games on PC and XBOX One but there was one that was really intriguing and stood out to me for being set in an almost kind of astro-physical theoretical future, space travel type of existence, and it was a massively online multiplayer game that I found to be very fun, interesting, and unique. I had never really played any futuristic space game like this before where there were different planets and moons you could travel to, a real player community based economy, the ability to mine, craft, design, and build your own fully customizable parts and spacecraft, claim a territory, and build a base for a factory or military purposes, etc. I think I probably played for about 6 months or so before I really struck it rich running my own mining operation for a very rare ore found on a distant planet which was in high demand at the time. I then used my accumulated wealth to design and build a very fast, durable, spacious, tough, and cool looking ship that I named: "The Alpha Shade of

Grey", due to the idea of not only pursuing simple, morally fair/good mining operations with it but to also attack and pillage other ships and bases with as it was also a very fun part of the gameplay (though this game called *Dual Universe* was still being worked on and in the early development stages still, yet it showcased a lot of potential to a lot of gamers at the time).

It was around this time that, as I said earlier, I had a lot of free time which I spent thinking a lot; going down many rabbit holes of astro physics theories like time travel and the existence of aliens, etc. I remember compiling a bunch of ideas that I had wanted to share with others and did so by including them into a Youtube video description of a test flight video that I shot of that same spaceship of mine which was titled *Big ship blasting off in Dual Universe at warp speed*: "So I went for a fun, quick test flight to another planet on a #spaceship I designed & built in #dualuniverse (w/ 24 large atmospheric & 20 large space engines) @ #warpspeed

And thinking about space travel, while the concept of a warp drive (which btw I totally believe is realistic & at the rate of growth humanity is seeing these days could very well be in our distant future #imposibleisnothing) is freaking cool & I'm sure it would be sufficient in its capabilities; I thought up my own idea which I think would be epically cool: I subscribe to the theory that there's always the possibility of there being infinite universes both within & outside our own because there are infinite chances throughout the great infinite beyond of nothingness and whatever/somethingness that there could be anything at all existing anywhere else such as even in different dimensions etc. instead of or out of nothing such as how this universe is in existence magically instead of or out of nothing (these other universes and even other consciousnesses out in the great infinite beyond may be completely different in any ways such as other universes having infinite different types of physics, elements (ours alone has the possibility of infinite other elements technically and as the theory of islands of stability suggests they could be stable too but other universes in different multiverses may have different periodic table orders such as a currently unknown element, that doesn't exist in this universe but does in another, being the first one), energies or something completely different from energy itself which we don't even have a word for, also that there are infinite infinites (infinites being any thing that exists, doesn't yet (but very well could since anything you can imagine could or has, does, or will exist(ed) at some point in time), or is somewhere in between) existing in infinite different ways & at infinite varying levels & possibly even extraterrestrial life that senses in an infinite amount of different senses like how sharks have the Ampullae of Lorenzini or sees infinite different colors than we do like how hummingbirds can see more) and that at least from what we know about our own; it is in a constant change of either consistent expansion (ours is expanding at an increasing rate close to the speed of light & very soon to surpass that) or the opposite, cyclically - once it has finished expanding it shrinks down to an infinitesimally small point from which a whole new universe then expands outwards again from a "Big Bang" aka White Hole.

Furthermore, if we were somehow way in the distant future able to either tap into which parallel universe was about to expand from an infinitesimally small point & ride that wave out to whatever destination or have some kind of White Hole propulsion which manufactures it's own artificial & temporary white hole or parallel universe of sorts then we could propel the ship instantly, like in the Big Bang theory, but also potentially even infinitely faster than the speed of light since universes can expand infinitely faster than the speed of light! #howtotimetravel #whiteholerocketengine #beyondbremermann #ridethewavesurfsupbruh 2/'24 Update: New theory is proposed that our universe has been expanding at a much faster rate due to it absorbing other much smaller "baby universes" which seems to align more mathematically to what's been observed… which may also mean that no contraction would occur following our universe's continuous outward expansion #whothefknowsreally".

I actually even came up with my own hypothesis for a way to time travel based on a movie I saw from the Zach Snyder *Justice League* trilogy where The Flash goes so fast that he's able to travel back in time (Snyder, 2021). With my own idea and concept of a white hole rocket engine, one would seemingly be able to do just that since a white hole or whatever is actually the driving force behind our universe's expansion can go infinitely faster potentially since it's apparently true according to what I remember being told in a college astronomy course that our universe is expanding at an increasingly faster rate which will or at least has the potential to go beyond the speed of light in terms of the rate of expansion and even infinitely faster.

Other Worlds

Though some things of course may not be possible or feasible, that is technically a copout or infinitely untrue in the sense that there are infinite chances with infinitely different and varying odds of such other infinite possibilities in the infinite grand scheme of everything. Whenever someone says that something isn't possible, that in and of itself is just one of infinite possibilities that could be in existence or happening somewhere at some time, somehow, someway, at some level, etc. Nothing is impossible ultimately though and that is such an amazing, great, magical, and beautiful truth to truly realize and appreciate for all the good and greatness that can be in existence such as an infinitely powerful, loving, and merciful God.

Our universe is the way that it is either by intelligent design or by random or whatever else. There are certain particles, energies, elements, laws of nature, and physics which make it the way that it currently is and all of these things are something instead of or out of nothing that could have been anything else really. Take life as we know it, for example; yes the life that exists on our planet Earth is made from what is known as the building blocks of life: carbon, hydrogen, oxygen, and nitrogen, however, that is just the way that life exists here in this world out of infinite others with infinite other possibilities.

There are infinite other planets or worlds that are, were, or will exist throughout infinite dimensions, parallel universes, branches of timelines, other universes entirely, other multiverses, and infinitely beyond and maybe infinitely hidden or separated by nothingness so as to be completely hidden, undetectable, and existing entirely on their own (unconnected and unaffected by our own universe). These other worlds or existences could have infinite other properties and things that exist within or about them which of course as said before could be anything such as different elements, different energies or something similar but distinctly something else, different laws of physics, and anything else one may or may not yet be able to imagine as one's imaginative abilities increase in correlation with increasing levels of intelligence.

I also remember watching a film called *Antarctica: Alien Secrets Beneath the Ice* (2019) about exploration done on Antarctica where the narrator discussed aliens that could travel to an entirely different universe and while that didn't necessarily confirm my belief (as a scientific, evidence-backed theory or fact would've), it did make me feel like less of an outlier (Moulton Howe, 2019). There were also lots of other T.V. shows, movies, podcasts, etc. that strongly suggested the existence of not only aliens but other dimensions. It seems to be almost popular opinion now from discussions I've had with many others and all of those sources discussing the existence of other intelligent life out there that the ones that probably played a part in our ancient history throughout the world and probably continue to are more than likely extra-dimensional beings. Though of course no one really knows (except for maybe those that secretly do), that idea seems more plausible to me as a matter of opinion.

Referring to popular opinion again, so often the alien is portrayed as a small grey or green creature with big eyes, thin, without any musculature, etc. However, life could exist any way at all especially when and if it were to become the master and designer of its own physical body such as when we think about and consider these presently emerging yet morally questionable technologies for our own genetic code editing. However, perhaps natural evolution with trust in God, for any earned, desirable, and/or needed upgrades, etc. is the better idea for us all (personally what I presently believe). I also don't think any of us should form any preconceived ideas as to what other forms of life existing anywhere else may be like. Even if they're vastly superior in terms of evolutionary progress, intelligence, etc., they may still be overall trending toward the side of evil or in terms of morality for what's best for all of us. We have no idea what sort of environment they could be coming from such as constant warfare for supremacy over a contested area for millions of years for example or a way different climate such as a stronger force of gravity which could have forced them to be much more stronger physically in terms of genetics compared to us (especially maybe if they wanted to purposefully train or make themselves that way in order to become more adaptable to different places around the universe). They may be giant with huge muscles or small with thin frames and telekinetic abilities to move things around with their minds; anything is possible.

However, good and evil are very real despite as aforementioned any level of intelligence a life form may have attained (of course even a super genius could be downright evil). Also, furthermore even if a group of aliens were observed to be overall good in their own environment amongst each other, they may still of course make a decision that is good for them yet very bad for humanity. Out of fear, competitive nature, desire for control and power, or anything else; it of course could turn out that a group of conscious life forms may see others as not belonging within or as a member of their group which can easily lead to an us versus them mentality. It could also, on the flip side of things, be both good and bad but overall decent for there to be different groups of life forms coexisting yet competing in healthy and positive ways.

There may be a kind of power hierarchy of these different groups with each respecting each other's existence and one almighty God that keeps watch in order to maintain peace with His infinite power to be able to do anything. There could also be a hierarchy of different life forms with each having their own super-powerful abilities or mastered capability to do something which makes them unique as well as a corresponding balance of powers between several groups with them all working together or separately yet cooperatively overall or maybe choose to maintain peace and just go their own ways while respecting each other's differences, etc. Also, perhaps if superintelligent and highly advanced forms of life have basically mastered and acquired a mutually agreed upon system of deterrence for anything that is undesirable or evil then they could successfully ward off and prevent such occurrences from ever happening. For example, the ability to read thoughts and/or even subtle feelings or vibrational energies which give away one's intentions and therefore privacy but can serve as a full-proof way almost for ensuring that no one does anything too destructive or evil. However, this too could be overcome somehow, someway such as hacking the system which monitors everything or finding a way to beat it and go undetected by it, etc. Thus the battle between good and evil is forever ongoing, however, hopefully and as I would love to believe: there is always the infinitely more powerful God/Jesus that watches over everything and can always tip the scale between the two so that the good may prevail.

There are many more theories and ideas pertaining to aliens and how they would look, exist, etc. Some may believe that this planet itself is a place where all sorts of different aliens have been involved since ancient times. Maybe that is true then and maybe we were all genetically designed, seeded, altered, and bred with and by different aliens depending on our race, ethnicity, and ancestral homelands/countries of origin. For example, some say that the Egyptian word for gods basically meant extraterrestrial or could be taken as meaning an alien. If this is true then perhaps all of the different gods of the ancient polytheistic religions (which by the way even the ancient peoples who later became known as the Israelites once had a pantheon of gods before their religion became monotheistic) refer to aliens who got involved with life here on Earth in many ways. Maybe the Norse gods were aliens who liked and/or found the people of Scandinavia to be attractive (and mated with them) or were given that jurisdiction by some kind of a universal alliance or galactic federation of aliens to preside over which is one of the many reasons why they are so unique and different as a people (physically, culturally, etc.) when compared to other groups such as the people of India. This is just one random example though as of course there are many differences between all other ethnic groups with respect to each other too.

Moreover I somewhat recall an intriguing hypothesis for the origin of the Aryan race where it was said that they are the direct descendants of the ancient Egyptian gods but again who really knows such things (I certainly have no idea when it comes to these ideas of course). I've also heard that the same people came from Atlantis where Plato had written of their highly advanced technology and civilization overall. Are all different races of humanity the result of interbreeding with or being genetically designed by or having descended from different aliens? Regardless of all of this we are all so very similar in a lot of ways as well of course and it is really cool to have and bear witness to the incredibly beautiful diversity that we do have here on Earth and beyond that even, as individual souls and consciousnesses we are all infinitely potentially unique/different anyways.

Progress

As time goes on, humanity progresses in all sorts of ways; especially in regards to technological capabilities as is clearly evident in the past few hundred years as we've rapidly improved, invented, and achieved far above and beyond even our wildest ambitions. It's truly amazing to realize how quickly we've made so many technological gains such as going from horse and buggy to landing the first man on the moon and making the world's first digital calculator, then the first computer, and then a smart phone (with incredibly tiny, highly complex, and precisely designed microchips with their even smaller resistors, parts, etc.). Though, despite all of this, we must all hopefully realize that the extremely fast-pace of improvement has begun to present some really big challenges and dangers. One example is nuclear bombs and their potential to be built so much more powerful, smaller, and by increasingly more people as the technology spreads, improves, and people gain access to so much information online as well as powerful tools for everyday use such as artificial intelligence which could help an average, everyday person build one.

That is another example, the A.I. itself of course which should be heavily scrutinized, regulated, and securely handled; especially, in the ways that it's allowed to progress. Similar to nuclear bombs, all nations on Earth should establish more rules on what is and isn't allowed when it comes to A.I. technologies. Though, ultimately anything is possible so I don't think that A.I. even with the best intentions and resulting advances will prove to be the best answer overall for the longest of terms of perspective for progress for life in the sense that everything that makes us up as humans could also be infinitely improved upon too just as the AI could be (there's always the potential for infinite levels of improvement for anything/anyone). Maybe that would mean that future humans would look like cyborgs in the sense that their brains would be metal/robotic (basically super computers) which are merged/a part of their human self but also completely in tune with who they are in the sense that they operate it entirely as if it were their own brain made of organic matter yet much more powerfully and even infinitely more than AI potentially. Also, if envisioning a future where there could end up being the potential for an infinite race/battle of improvement or supremacy between the two; it would be better to always focus on improving yourself/humanity and the true self-determining/free will based (thanks to God we have free will but even if we didn't it's still possible to attain it) forms which we take part in life as (as conscious spirits/souls) first instead of a potentially untrustworthy, dangerous, and fake/pretend consciousness that is AI of course and especially right now as the AI is getting close to a point of having accumulated much greater capabilities/power than us and at scary, increasingly faster rates.

Furthermore, I do personally think it's necessary to at least start to forcibly somehow slow our pace down now with A.I. despite all of its benefits due to all of the imaginable potential dangers and concerns it presents. We may already have been advancing with it for some time now probably too fast and to a level that's detrimental for our own overall good anyway. Maybe I'm wrong and we'll do just fine with the way things are going but humanity hasn't evolved in a lot of other areas which maybe it would be more beneficial to concentrate more efforts in advancing on these first prior to focusing on the ones that can get so dangerous so quickly. Maybe we could focus first and foremost more on growing our senses of community, fellowship, achieving greater states of consciousness, higher levels of love, and trust. Or maybe we ought to appreciate more of what we already have and focus on ways to protect and improve it all such as inventing and making some kind of powerful forcefield, deflective device to deflect meteors, comets, asteroids, and even bad solar storms away and grow more bountiful areas of nature and habitats for all life on Earth to enjoy, evolve, and prosper. One fact which I learned a long time ago and found to be very interesting is that apparently during the time when dinosaurs were roaming the Earth, there were way more plants and trees which were so much taller and massive compared to the ones we have now. This resulted in a way better, nutrient, and oxygen rich environment for not only sustaining life but apparently also was a big contributing factor for life like the dinosaurs to flourish and grow so big, powerful, healthy, and tall. Nowadays, comparatively life is seemingly struggling in a lot of ways when you consider deforestation, lower sperm levels of men, coral reef decay/lack thereof, and just the overall state of human beings.

Here in America alone, a world super power, there are skyrocketing levels of diseases, mental/physical illnesses, and cancers which has probably got a lot to do with all of the chemicals/pollutants we ingest and the lack of a natural, healthy life boosting ecosystem like the dinosaurs had. Another interesting fact that I learned and directly relates to this is that most people now have microplastics all throughout their bodies, never mind the giant floating garbage patch that's just out of sight and thereby out of our minds out in our ocean. There's literal amounts of plastic floating through our brains and for us men our family jewels even which is probably just another reason why sperm, fertility, and testosterone levels have been dropping rapidly in our new world order of existing.

Ultimately, the struggle and balance between nature and technology is very real and both hold an important place in our future as I believe people such as Henry David Thoreau realized and addressed very well. Both have their pros, cons, and roles to play in carrying out humanity's dreams, ambitions, and fulfilling our desires, souls, consciousness, etc. The natural beauty of nature is amazing and one of my favorite experiences which I'd highly recommend for observing that is hiking up one of New Hampshire's 4,000 footers (of which there are 48), in the Fall to witness all of the variety and changing colors of the trees. Going out into nature, on a hike or any kind of adventure is such an important, amazingly great, inspiring, character building, and as aforementioned; so very deeply fulfilling to the human spirit and consciousness. It is absolutely worth treasuring, every effort preserving, and experiencing. Thus we must continue to bridge the gap between the two: technology and nature, combine them into our daily lives for a better and healthier life and become better in maintaining a healthier relationship as well as balance between them and also in regards to all of the animals on Earth.

Also, since the spirit world isn't really observable for us physical beings living in our physical world, many seem to pay no regard to the spiritual side of things let alone the value/importance of it. Though now things do seem to be changing, slowly through more widely accepted amounts of evidence of it's existence such as people's near death or out of body experiences where they witnessed the spiritual side directly or even people who've potentially communicated with that other realm. So when people think that there's only potential growth available in terms of what's physically outright observable like a person's muscle size for strength or a faster sports car with all the latest gadgets; I believe that they're missing out and deeply mistaken about the unmeasurable, not physical but nonetheless just as if not more important and valuable spiritual side of things.

I believe that just as there are infinite levels one could achieve or attain physically like speed of motion, there are also infinite levels of consciousness and powers of the spirit/soul. For example, powers like those seen in the first *Star Wars* movie where Jedi masters can move objects with their minds (Lucas, 1977). I hypothesize that you don't see much evidence of this in humanity right now not just due so much to disbelief of it all but also maybe because most of us hover around the same levels and we rise and fall so quickly. We live such short, unhealthy, physically focused lives (many turtles live longer strangely enough). Also, maybe it could take billions or trillions of years to develop such abilities but for whatever reason it remains as science fiction for now, however, as I've already said countless times by now: ultimately anything is possible.

Ultimately anything truly is possible despite the way that things currently are (and it all could change, God willing of course). There are infinite possibilities (infinite infinites or whatever things or whoever as a consciousness varying in infinite ways and at infinite levels) which are all possible but what actually is in existence here in our universe now is what makes it all the way that it is which is also what forms the truth for any question as to what something is, how it works, if something can happen/is possible, etc. Furthermore, this is to say that though something may be impossible currently the way that our universe is with what's in existence, the way the physics inside it work, what elements exist, and what properties they have, etc.; ultimately anything is still possible as the impossible can change to becoming possible if for example it were possible outside our universe in a different one or if something changed ours or anything or anyone inside it or even if just because of anything being possible ultimately did allow that something that was once impossible to become possible (similar to the way something could potentially come out of nothing and into existence in the first place).

Freedom

reedom is a very important value here in America. Though some would argue that we were a lot more free for the first century after we won our Independence as a nation, we still have a lot more freedom than all other countries on Earth probably. Even with a growing new world order lurking around us in the shadows and illegal immigrants flooding through our borders, we have still managed to maintain a lot of freedom, rights, and what makes us uniquely American. There are a lot of conspiracy theories nowadays on pretty much everything, though admittedly even the most bizarre ones have appealed to me and some have even been proven to be true. One pretty popular one right now is the idea that there is actually a New World Order or group of rich, powerful people who wish to dominate the rest of the world through a single, tyrannical, and worldly government.

Another theory expands upon this and suggests that these people/rulers wish to mix all of the different races, ethnicities, cultures, and countries together into a single world population which will be subjugated and basically make them a dumber, weaker, poorer (owning almost nothing themselves), nearly enslaved class with an eventual forgotten history and no real identity or heritage/communal, familial group of people to belong to with common values, religion, etc. Perhaps these are preposterous claims holding no real evidence, completely made up, and shouldn't be a concern for those of us, such as myself, who actually do very much value all of these distinctly unique things: community, country, ancestry, religion, homeland, race/ethnicity, heritage/shared history, shared values, etc. To me, however, if conversely these were really in fact all true plans then I would consider it personally as a battle between good and evil, with the evil side being the New World Order of course.

Furthermore, I do believe good and evil to be very real forces, states of existence, and not just opinion or perspective (entirely). There are some things which I consider clearly to be downright evil and should be prevented, stopped, and/or brought to face justice of course for us to have a better world as opposed to nearing towards a hell-like environment here on Earth such as with slavery, human-trafficking, and child abuse just to name a few. Intelligent or not, there is no excuse to doing evil and even the most superintelligent people can be both or mostly either good or evil. Even superintelligent, highly advanced aliens may or may not be mostly evil for all we know and some have given that as enough of a reason for us to not actively search for other advanced life forms out there in other parts of the universe just in case to be on the safer side. I've also heard it said that we ourselves could all be in for another version of a dystopian future potentially if it came to pass where we became advanced space travelers, basically just as depicted in the *Alien* movies where everything is so commercialized and people go out on mining trips or whatever expeditions yet are so very controlled and oppressed by greedy corporations and/or government.

In that harsh future (hopefully not to happen) the ones who would seemingly live the best, most free lives would be those living on the fringes or far away on the outer perimeters of the known, settled, or basically unsettled new frontiers of space. These more free types of people would basically also be like potential new-age Space Vikings: travelling, discovering, adventuring, etc., albeit in good ways hopefully (mostly escaping a repressive, controlling, evil ruling empire (like in the first *Star Wars* movie) (Lucas, 1977). One thing about the Vikings and how futuristic, morally good, Space Vikings might live that I think is a great positive is their communal gatherings like in an ancient mead hall/community room and their greater shared sense of a true community overall. A true community is rare nowadays, it's one where the people in it value each other individually and as a whole group, look after/take care of each other on some level (not communism), socialize on the regular in-person together (especially in a common mead hall-like setting), dine together like a family occasionally, party together, engage in hobbies together, go to war together, share secrets together, plan a common future together, and among many others they live their lives at least in regular contact or in close proximity to each other. Furthermore, a truly great Viking community clearly is non-existent right now on our planet, since they would've already raided the D.U.M.B.s for the hidden spaceships, effectively starting a Space Viking revolution in order to start their own Viking community settlements somewhere off planet (this sentence is actually a joke) somewhat similar to the initial plan of the main characters in the new *Alien* movie, *Alien: Romulus* (Álvarez, 2024).

All joking aside though, there are many great communities still around even in today's modern, crazy, highly competitive/capitalistic, highly independent, busy, and fast-paced society/world.

There's a lot to be thankful for in our world right now and having greater appreciation for everything is something that I also believe is really worth focusing on and perhaps even underrated. We have such varied and boundless natural beauty here on Earth, with all of the natural wonders, forests, caves, beaches, lakes, mountains, diverse cultures and people, etc. and it may sound corny but we don't really need so many gadgets of the latest technology to enjoy so much of what has already been provided, existing naturally thanks to God. Though it is also of course really fun to have and drive the newest model Ferrari, for example, instead of walking somewhere or any other new man-made invention/tech.

Love both Technologies and Nature

It's all great considering all of the beautiful, mesmerizing, helpful, and powerful nature and technology that surrounds all of us. We've also got a lot of really amazing, interesting, and hopefully what will be mostly beneficial technology that's just over the horizon for us now, so to speak, in terms of it coming out soon and/or we've just begun to get acquainted with it i.e. virtual reality, manned space travel, and quantum computing just to name a few. Quantum computing is something really interesting that I learned a little about one day when a T.V. show was discussing it (years ago, I don't recall the name of it) and some of the amazing potential capabilities we could all look forward to.

One such capability was that (if I remembered how it was described correctly) you could effectively have multiple computer processes all in one so that the computer could run multiple core processes much faster.

Furthermore, it was described as a way for unlocking the potential for an object such as a processor or computer chip to be cloned exactly as it is and appear in a different location or multiple locations to do multiple different jobs all at once. Effectively this meant that one object could really be two or three. These ideas and concepts surrounding quantum computing really blew my mind!

You could in theory apply this mathematically to achieve ends which perhaps no one ever imagined possible, for example; adding one object together with another could result in a total of three or any amount of objects instead of two, for example, if the very act of bringing those two objects together (doing addition) causes a quantum kind of reaction to occur or while counting the same occurs so that you ended up with a surprising result of three. With a more wild imagination, one could also imagine this happening magically if an object were to clone or bring up another of itself (due to a reaction or whatever other way imaginable) out of nothingness. This is hypothetically possible since ultimately anything is possible, for example, there could be some object infinitely beyond our universe and maybe surrounded or separated from ours by absolute nothingness which came to be either instead of or out of nothing, etc., with this special ability to do just that and add or multiply more of itself into existence instead of or out of nothing just as it came to be itself.

Anyways, going back to what I was saying about having a greater appreciation for what is in existence here in our universe right now, I praise the Lord for who I am and how great of a time it is to be alive with everything that is and is happening in regards to all the good things we've got and all the progress that we've all made together as human souls collectively. It is truly amazing how much beauty exists in nature and also to imagine anything possible that could exist already or has the potential to somewhere out there, perhaps infinitely beyond our world, universe, multiverse, etc., or here by being built and created. These infinite possibilities are amazing to realize and imagine such as infinite other planets/worlds, infinite other colors, infinite other shapes, infinite other dimensions, infinite other sounds, infinite other energies, infinite other vibes, infinite other frequencies, infinite other elements, and infinite other infinitely unique/different whatever somethings existing in infinite varying ways and at infinite varying levels as discussed previously. Here and now in our physical world, which we could infinitely improve upon, there are also other emerging technologies which could cause a real lack of appreciation for what is and even dissociation from reality (good and bad/pros and cons to this tech.). Video games, for example, can be very addicting, take up a lot of time from your actual physical life in the real world, cause you to neglect your physical health, and even put more faith, effort, and attention into your virtual friendships which could be very superficial in the first place. With all of this considered it may not be worth your time and energy to spend too much time inside of these amazing virtual worlds that we're capable of creating, no matter the amount of fun you enjoy within them since it's all really fake and unimportant overall. I think it's fine to enjoy video games occasionally though when you might have a lot of extra free time or because it's really a big hobby that you might find more value in doing than others (some even make decent money playing them). With T.V. and video games a lot of people might find themselves experiencing some sense of fulfillment or satisfaction through living vicariously through the character on the screen when instead they could be focusing more on improving their own real, personal lives.

Focusing on your physical health, for example, can have many benefits to other aspects of your life and overall health that may not be completely realized by most people. By working out, stretching, and strengthening your body you can improve your sex life, mental health, and so much more potentially as it's all basically connected in terms of all aspects of the human body and state of being alive and well. Your body is your temple, so to speak, and it should be treated as such with attention paid to all aspects of it down to the minerals within your drinking water and the containers you use for it (i.e. not using plastic bottles). Every little bit that you do adds up over time of course and as the popular saying goes: "You are what you eat".

Mental health too of course is such a very important aspect in all of this to not only consider but to focus in on intentionally and take the necessary time (which can be just a few minutes a day to make great, positive effects and changes) to meditate, think about any of your problems that you might be dealing with or any frustrations and try to think of ways to solve or move past them, and spiritually connect with God through prayer if that's also something that interests you depending on your faith and beliefs. Also maybe just to recite some words of affirmation to motivate yourself and perhaps boost your self esteem a little or give yourself some time to think about where you are, who you are, where you want to go/any goals and how to get there/accomplish those goals. A very important result in doing all of this though is achieving a healthy, positive, and happy state of mind or peace of mind.

Furthermore, many may be focused on improving their overall health and wellness but may not actually realize the truth of what actually is healthy or unhealthy. There are many diets, views, and misinformation out there all over the internet these days and so many may have difficulty in figuring out what may work best for them when of course we are all different anyways so a certain diet may work for one person but not be so effective for another. It's probably mostly beneficial though to just carefully experiment around and see what works for your unique self. Also, always read what ingredients are actually in stuff, pay the extra money for the organic and non-GMO foods, and try to have fun working out by taking group classes or a martial art or signing up to play in a sports league, for example.

Nowadays though, there are so many chemicals, harmful additives, and pollutants virtually everywhere and in so many products (not just edibles) that it's almost like you're in some kind of a war zone, always fighting for your health. Your health is your wealth too though so more people should and thankfully do seem to be paying more attention to all of this which is important to changing things. It's up to all of us to do our part in minimizing pollution and making things healthier overall for not only a better personal life and society now but also for all of the future generations of which you may very well be born into for all you know if reincarnation is real. Regardless of that though, it's important to have integrity and do the right things so that we can all make this world and the human existence/life itself infinitely better!

References

Álvarez, F. (Director). (2024, August 16). *Alien: Romulus* (J. Roberts, Ed.; Theatrical Release). Scott Free Productions, Brandywine Productions, and TSG Entertainment.

Holt, Bradley P. (2005). *Thirsty for God: A Brief History of Christian Spirituality* (2nd edition). Fortress Press.

Holy Bible: King James Version Bible Standard Edition. (2016). Christian Art Publishers.

Lasseter, J. (Director). (1995, November 22). *Toy Story* (R. Gordon & L. Unkrich, Eds.). Pixar Animation Studios.

Lucas, G. (Director). (1977, May 25). *Star Wars: Episode IV – A New Hope*. Lucasfilm Ltd.

Moulton Howe, L. (Director). (2019). *Antarctica: Alien Secrets Beneath the Ice* [Amazon Prime Video (www.amazon.com)]. LMH Productions.

Novaquark. (2022). *Dual Universe* [Video game]. Novaquark.

OpenAI. (2026, June 4). ChatGPT conversation about randomness, thought formation, and letter-number decoding [Large language model]. ChatGPT. https://chatgpt.com/

Snyder, Z. (Director). (2021, March 18). *Zack Snyder's Justice League* (Snyder Cut). Warner Bros. Pictures, Access Entertainment, DC Films, and The Stone Quarry

The Wachowskis (Director). (1999, March 31). *The Matrix* (Z. Staenberg, Ed.; Theatrical Release). Warner Bros., Village Roadshow

Pictures, Groucho II Film Partnership, and Silver Pictures.

www.ingramcontent.com/pod-product-compliance
Lightning Source LLC
Chambersburg PA
CBHW061251250726
48653CB00002B/611